# The Future of Mankind

## As Related to Food Chemistry

John Kayvanfar, MD

iUniverse, Inc.
Bloomington

The Future of Mankind
As Related to Food Chemistry

The information, ideas, and suggestions in this book are not intended
as a substitute for professional medical advice. Before following any
suggestions contained in this book, you should consult your personal
physician. Neither the author nor the publisher shall be liable or responsible
for any loss or damage allegedly arising as a consequence of your use
or application of any information or suggestions in this book.

iUniverse books may be ordered through booksellers or by contacting:

iUniverse
1663 Liberty Drive
Bloomington, IN 47403
www.iuniverse.com
1-800-Authors (1-800-288-4677)

Because of the dynamic nature of the Internet, any Web addresses or
links contained in this book may have changed since publication and
may no longer be valid. The views expressed in this work are solely those
of the author and do not necessarily reflect the views of the publisher,
and the publisher hereby disclaims any responsibility for them.

Any people depicted in stock imagery provided by Thinkstock are models,
and such images are being used for illustrative purposes only.

Certain stock imagery © Thinkstock.

ISBN: 978-1-4759-1131-2 (sc)
ISBN: 978-1-4759-1133-6 (e)

Library of Congress Control Number: 2012916321

Printed in the United States of America

iUniverse rev. date: 10/1/2012

# Acknowledgments

My appreciation to my family who, allowed me to take valuable time from their life, to write this book.

# Contents

# Introduction

*I have gathered the material in this book from my years of medical education, experiences during the practice of medicine, and further research.*

We all learn from knowledge of the past and continue to improve upon it. What we are practicing today in medicine is one way to look at things, but this book will clear your mind on some of the questions that you may have. It will provide another way of looking at health problems and their solutions in medicine.

I have been in the practice of medicine and orthopedic surgery in Southern California for twenty-six years.

This book is about *my own observation of changes* that I have noticed in my practice of orthopedics and medicine in terms of disease conditions and the problems humans have been experiencing and will be facing for years to come; these problems will not get better, but worse with time. This does not seem to be just in Southern California. From talking to my colleagues from around the nation, it seems to be true in all parts of the United States. This seems also to be happening in other countries around the globe.

I was always in love with science and medicine. I have always used my education to better help my patients. Through continuous observation and treatment of my patients, I have noticed that certain diseases and conditions are on the rise, so I have tried to find a solution as well as a treatment for their problems. Being a family man, I have seen many young adults that are also affected. My son, through his education as a biomedical engineering major has educated me on how our body repairs itself.

My sincere wish is that by educating people, collectively we can make some positive changes in our approach to healthier life.

# Chapter One

## Disease Central: Where We Are Today

### How It All Started

A few years into my practice, about twenty-two years ago, one of my patients walked in to be seen. After the usual greetings, she stated, "Doctor, I am here because the numbness and pain in my hand are back and are getting worse." She reminded me, I performed carpal tunnel surgery on her wrist three years earlier. She stated was doing fine until a year ago. After taking her history and examining her neck and upper extremities, including the hands, her complaint was confirmed.

I scratched my head and told her that in orthopedic books, carpal tunnel syndrome is generally considered to be a compression neuropathy. In other words, the pain is caused by direct pressure on the nerve. Since her surgery would have relieved that pressure, I had no other recommendation for her at the time. Therefore, I made the following suggestion: I asked my patient to give me three weeks to come up with an idea for her and get to the bottom of the problem. Maybe then we could come with answers to solve her problem or problems.

The next three weeks became a project for me to solve her problem.

My analysis went as follows: Compression neuropathy by definition means a nerve is pressed on by external forces—in this case, deep transverse carpal ligament or tendons within the carpal tunnel space, which is not an expandable space. Since she already under went carpal tunnel surgery, her problem could not be considered just a compression neuropathy anymore. This meant either the nerve had developed edema and was pressing against the ligament or tendons, which are harder structures than the nerve is; or the ligament had developed edema or inflammation and was pressing against the nerve, the softer structure. Or perhaps both had happened, with problems in both the nerve and tendons, which caused both inflammation and edema. Either way, something was swelling or was inflamed. There could be no other scenario.

This meant we were dealing with neuropathy and not solely compression neuropathy. Probably other components were involved (meaning the nerve was not able to do its job right because of other factor or factors). My goal became to determine what was the cause of inflammation or edema. In this case, another surgery would not do her any good.

Since the first two scenarios were old and surgery should have helped permanently, the fact that her problem was coming back meant the theory of compression neuropathy was no longer viable. Therefore only the third theory (internal problem/ neuropathy) was plausible.

I went back to basics and reviewed the literature, looking for all possible causes of neuropathy. The most common problems that cause carpal tunnel syndrome are thyroid problems, diabetes, and autoimmune disorders. After putting the list together, I designed a series of blood tests to detect those conditions.

When my patient came back for follow-up, I discussed my plan with her. She told me she had been to four other doctors and no one had any ideas for her. She agreed with the plan, stating, "At least you have a plan that might work." She agreed to go ahead and have the blood tests that I had chosen to be done.

After the test results came back, the results were discussed with her. Surprisingly all her results were normal according to the lab standard. To test for thyroid problems, you check for thyroid-stimulating hormone, T3 and T4 (T3 and T4 are different components of thyroid hormones). Her TSH was 5.0, which according to the lab standard was normal (normal was between 0.3 and 5.5). Could it be that the guidelines were incorrect? After obtaining more careful history and examination of the patient again, I found she had other aches and pain. She said, "Those are routine pains, and I am getting used to them." I also noticed she had some tender tendons. With that in mind, I analyzed hormone values cannot really have such a wide range of normality. My experience from medical school days and looking at the results of TSH in normal people showed that a normal value was always below 2.0. The scenario was discussed with her, and she agreed to try thyroid medication to bring the TSH to below 2.0.

Four weeks later, she was seen again. Her hand pain and numbness were much improved, but some numbness was persisting. Lab testing was done again for TSH, which was 1.6. After two months had passed, the numbness was still there and not improving to normal level.

Could it be that there was some sort of deficiency going on? We reviewed her diet, which was an average American diet. Then we did blood tests on vitamins that could cause neuropathy. Again the results came back normal, but at the lower limit of normal on B6, B12, and folic acid. I suggested to her to take small but specific doses of vitamins (B6 = 50mg, B12 = 500mcg, and folic acid = 800mcg/day).

A month later, she came in smiling and stated her numbness was going away and she felt normal again.

Since then, I have cut down on surgery for carpal tunnel syndrome from five or six per week to two or three per year. Almost all of my patients are being treated with medicines (*without surgery*) after finding the underlying problems. Patients recover to normal without residual problems. The only patients who need surgery are the ones whose problems have been going on for *a few years* without any treatment for the underlying cause, and thus they have developed muscle atrophy.

I wondered if the normal values could be wrong for some other tests too. Normal values are decided by getting a group of people together and, through questionnaires, asking if anything is wrong with them. If not, then their values are decided to be normal according to a bell-shaped curve. Were the normal numbers wrong, or was something else going on?

Since for years people were doing well, all the lab values could not be wrong. Could it be that for some reasons, the threshold for developing problems was changing because something was causing the body not be able to do proper repair processing? Or is there something wrong with food, which is preventing proper repair process?

With the above in mind, I kept seeing this kind of problem more and more as time went on.

Once I even saw a patient with AVN (avascular necrosis, where the ball of the hip joint becomes a dead tissue in the body, which causes arthritis and hip pain) with severe hypothyroidism (TSH of 25). After treatment of hypothyroidism, the avascular necrosis stopped and the pain stopped. An X-ray showed that the hip condition had improved. That told me a bit more about the function of the thyroid in the body. This meant it also works on the capillary endothelial wall of arteriole blood vessels (the smallest blood vessels, which are very small pipes, which take blood to the tissues). It also improves the blood flow to tissues all over the body (including bones). All tissues in the body are live and need oxygen and nutrients continuously. If the brain does not get them, you are brain dead.

We have been seeing more similar problems, other autoimmune disorders, and metabolic problems in patients than we have ever seen before. Their number is on the rise, and nowhere in the history of medicine have the frequency and prevalence been documented.

Normal values should not and can be decided on mathematical basis.

## Common Health Problems

What health problems have been happening to people?

*Obesity* is on the rise, and more people, including children, are gaining weight at an alarming rate.

More people experience *foot pain* at the bottom of the foot without any trauma.

More people experience *ankle or heel pain—or both*—without any trauma.

Increasingly people experience *knee pain* or so called osteoarthritis at younger age without any trauma.

More and, more people experience *hip pain or arthritis at young age* without any trauma.

Increasingly people experience *lower back pain and arthritis* without any trauma.

More and more people experience *neck or upper back pain* without any trauma or injury.

Increasingly people are *not able to sleep*, in spite of having active lives.

More and more people are developing *infections of all types*.

Increasingly people are developing *aches and pains, so-called fibromyalgia*, without any explanation.

Some people have problems that start with pain in their thigh, calf, or leg. Such as a woman shown on an ABC television morning news program last year (seen by me that eventually lost one of her legs).

The rate of *cancer* is on the rise.

We are seeing more and more people with *dry eye*.

Increasingly children are born affected by conditions that affect the brain, like *ADHD, mental retardation,* and *autism,* and become dependent on adults and eventually on society.

## Common (but Unsatisfactory) Treatments

What is happening now?

We are increasingly seeing patients with neck pain, shoulder pain, arm pain, and hand pain, with numbness and tingling, either in upper or lower extremities.

We are also seeing more and more people with low back pain, hip pain, leg pain, and foot and ankle pain.

The pain starts in one place or the other and very slowly goes to other parts of the body. In fact, before twenty years ago, we never saw anyone with chronic muscular-skeletal or body pain.

I am seeing more patients with muscular-skeletal (joint and muscle) *pain.* The number of patients with chronic pain has been continuously on the rise. I never saw such a high number of patients with chronic pain before twenty-five years ago, not even in my residency programs, which took seven years. Now we know *Chronic pain, in joints,* is the consequence of inflammation and eventually causes arthritis at any age.

*Let us see what type of treatment you are offered now.*

You visit your primary care doctor. He gives you an anti-inflammatory medicine, such as Naprosyn (also known as anaprox or Aleve), Motrin or ibuprofen, or Voltaren (also known as diclofenac), as well as prescription pain medication. You may also receive some anti-inflammatory creams.

You take this for a while. It may work for a while or not work. It helps some with the pain, because all NSAIDs (anti-inflammatory medicine) have painkilling effect.

Next, you see an orthopedist for treatment. Even some of the best diagnose you with sprain and strain with no history of trauma or any injury. You receive a prescription for another anti-inflammatory, stronger pain medication, plus a muscle relaxant (Flexeril = cyclobenzaprine, Skelaxin = metaxalone, Robaxin = methocabamol, or Soma = carisopprodol). You may also receive therapy. This also helps temporarily, but eventually will fail.

Then you are recommended to have surgery on your hand for carpal tunnel syndrome, surgery for Cubital tunnel syndrome, surgery for a Radial tunnel, or surgery on your shoulder or your neck and back. You feel a little better for a while. But you expected more relief. Then you get more therapy and maybe stronger pain medications. Maybe you receive ultrasonic treatment for lateral Epicondylitis (tennis elbow) or plantar fasciitis. You may even get steroids or injections too. All will work for a while.

For *back pain,* you get the same. If you have a reasonably normal MRI, you are referred for steroid injection or acupuncture and finally to pain management.

If your MRI shows some degenerative changes, then you are recommended to have more therapy. When it does not work, you are asked to have surgery.

If you have *knee pain* and developing arthritis, then it is read as degenerative joint disease by a radiologist and you are offered surgery like arthroscopic surgery on your knee.

Most doctors do not think you are too young to develop arthritis, or why are you developing it?

Most doctors do not come up with the question "Why are you developing obesity?"

Eventually you are offered multiple surgeries, and at the end, there is a total knee replacement.

When it comes to a point that regular pain medications do not work anymore, then you are referred directly to pain management.

Why? The treatment above is offered because; it is the standard of care (in other words, the treatment generally accepted as proper medical care within the medical community).

Interestingly with orthopedists or even other doctors, you are diagnosed with sprain and strain with no history of any kind of injury. This treatment for chronic pain is so common that doctors believe it is sprain and strain. Sometimes this therapy business goes on for months, without any or much permanent benefit.

It is also common practice to advise diet and exercise, diet and exercise, even in the media. In private meetings, some doctors are quite honest and admit we do not know what is happening.

# Chapter Two

## The Root Of The Problems

### What the Human Body Needs

In order for us to live, we humans need to have available *healthy food*. This is due to the fact that *our existence depends on what we consume*, whether it is "solid" or "liquid" in nature. In order to make this matter simpler to understand, imagine if you use cheap, and not clean, *gas* in your car. Your car engine eventually will break down because the injectors will not stay clean. The same goes for the human body. As a matter of fact, our body is much more *sensitive*, precise, *complicated*, and *complex* than our car.

## A little Biology

The human body is made up of millions of cells that must be in coexistence and harmony with each other all over the body. Every large group of cells is arranged to do specific tasks. These groups of cells are called *organs*. During the development phase of the fetus, certain groups of cells became the brain, nervous system, eyes, and bones. Other cell groups became the heart, lung, liver, fat, stomach, intestine, bone marrow, immune system, and skin. All organs need to work *in harmony* and without malfunction. If one organ (group of cells) stops working correctly, it will affect other groups of cells (organs). For example, if your heart stops beating and does not pump blood to other systems, we all know what the outcome is. You die. Why? Because all cells need oxygen and nutrients to survive. This arrives to them via the blood. The heart pumps blood to all organs, which consist of many cells.

Humans, like other living things, need specific food products as nutrition not only to live, but also to survive. Our body lives and survives from nutrition by repairing itself. Those who grew up during my time and watched the television series *Star Trek* know Mr. Spock used to say we are biological units. Biological units need to repair themselves by specific organic chemical materials, which *was originally available* on the planet earth, called *food*. These materials that we call *food* have nutrients that consist of very exact *chemistry*.

## A Bit about Food Chemistry

Imagine that you are looking at a chair with a specific shape and looking at another chair with another shape. Both are chairs, but they have two different shapes and sizes.

The shape of the two chairs and their sizes are very important elements in chemistry and they make the difference in chemistry between two different chairs. A small chair can fit under a small table or go through a small door, but a larger one cannot.

A simpler way to present this is to imagine children playing with LEGO pieces (cubes and triangles). The different pieces need to be the exact size and shape to fit into their corresponding slot in the cube. The bigger cubes, for example, will not fit into the slot of the small one.

In our body, it is not only similar, but much more complicated.

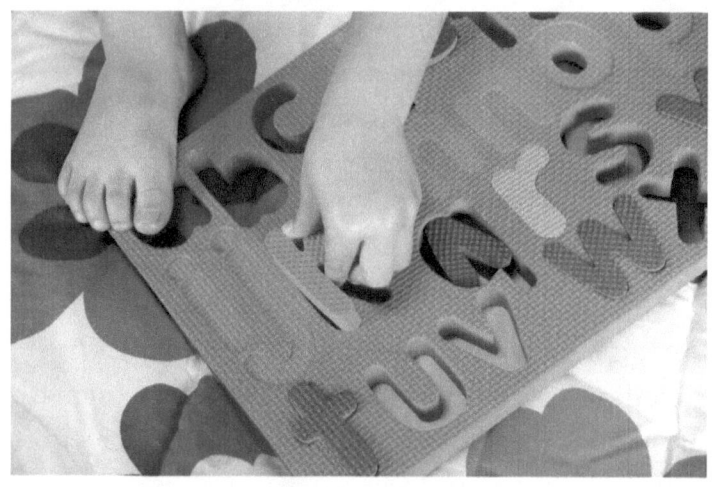

Each piece fits in their own slot only

Imagine your child is playing with a puzzle that has a specific picture on it. The picture is cut into many pieces. There are many rectangular pieces, for example, that are the same size. The one that fits into the appropriate place in the picture puzzle is the one that corresponds with the rest of the picture or image.

Pieces need to fit

Now to make matters more complicated, a puzzle is two-dimensional in play, but in a body, the puzzle is three-dimensional.

This means your body can only use the exact material or nutrients or food it needs in *exact chemistry*. Our body in one way or another will reject any similar shape or structure that is not exactly the chemistry we need. If it does not get what it needs, the body machine will finally breakdown in the form of conditions or diseases.

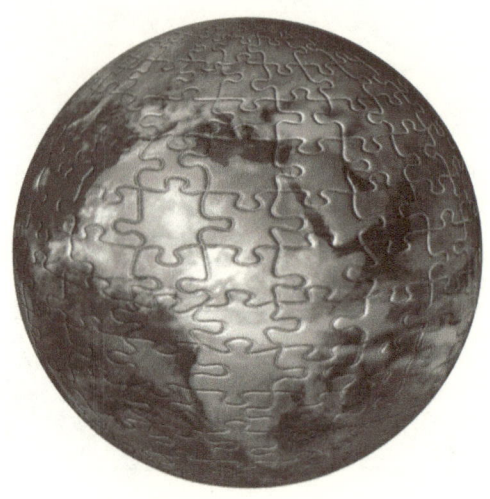

Unless pieces are in proper places,
you will not end up with a globe
picture on the surface of the ball

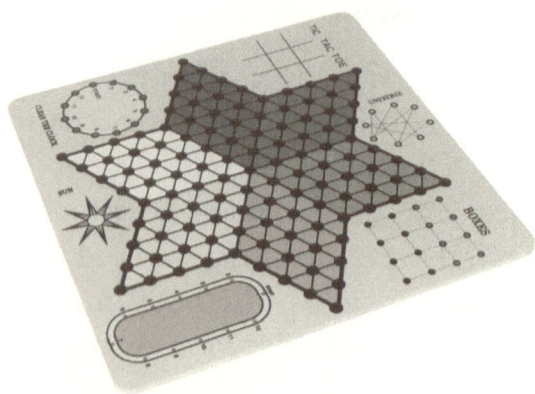

Unless color and lines and pieces are
in proper places, you will not end up
with accurate and colors and stars

To make matters even more complicated, the repair process in the body is done through a process called RNA transcription. Imagine a factory is making parts for a car. It needs to pour hot liquid metal into molds to make parts. Your body is almost similar, except that there is no solid mold in the body. Molds in the body are formed (made) by a specific live structure, called a *gene* that can process food to create different exact chemicals for the body to repair itself. These different molds are alive and use the same exact chemicals to live and stay alive themselves. These structures or body parts or genes repair our body by making different chemicals to repair the body as a whole (all organs).

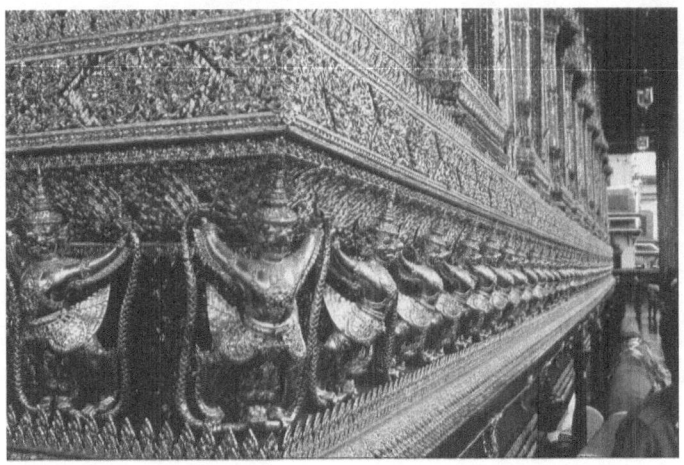

Without proper molding, you will not manufacture correct pieces of machinery

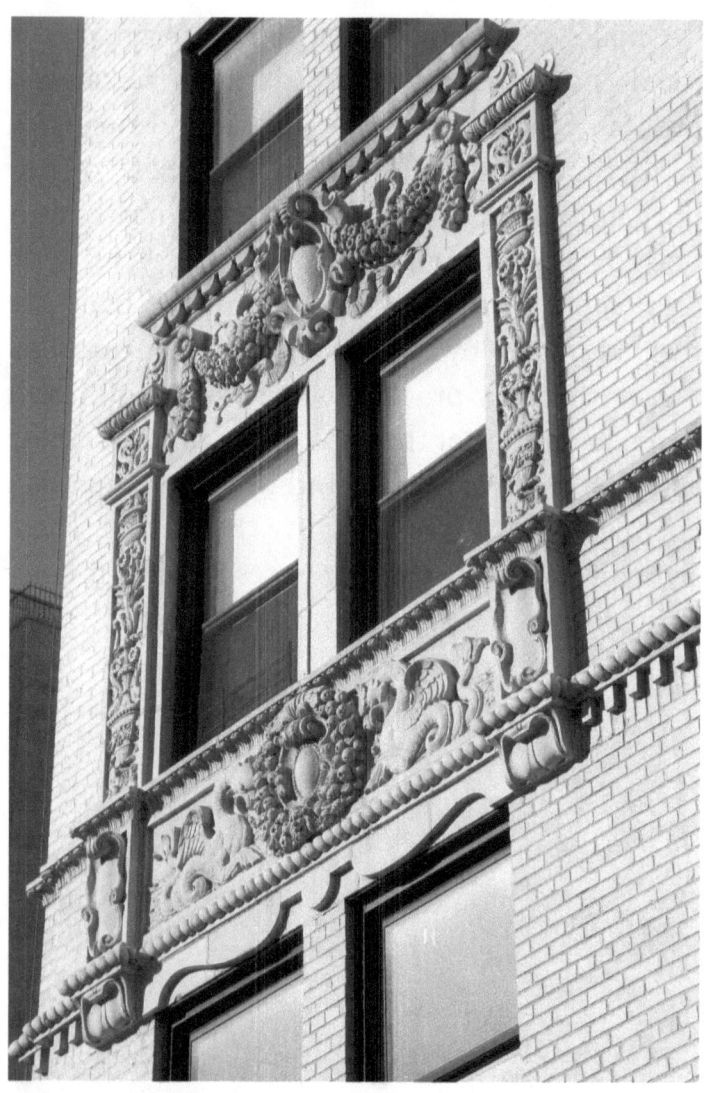

Without proper carving, you do not
end up with this beautiful product

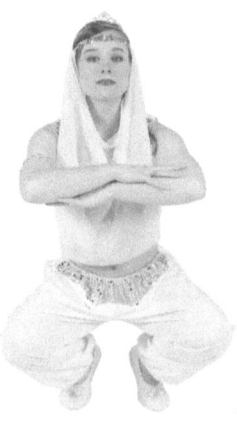

Unless all chemistry (all components=all pieces of puzzle) are correct chemistry, one will not be able to see this end product in this picture

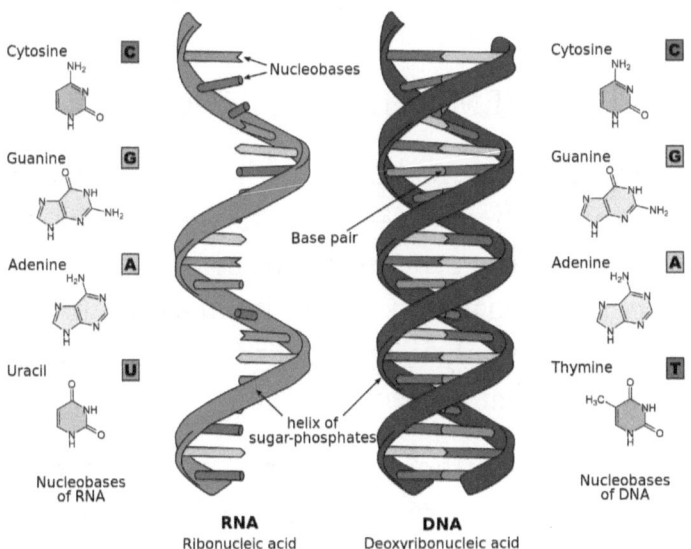

# DNA AND RNA IN SIMPLE FORM

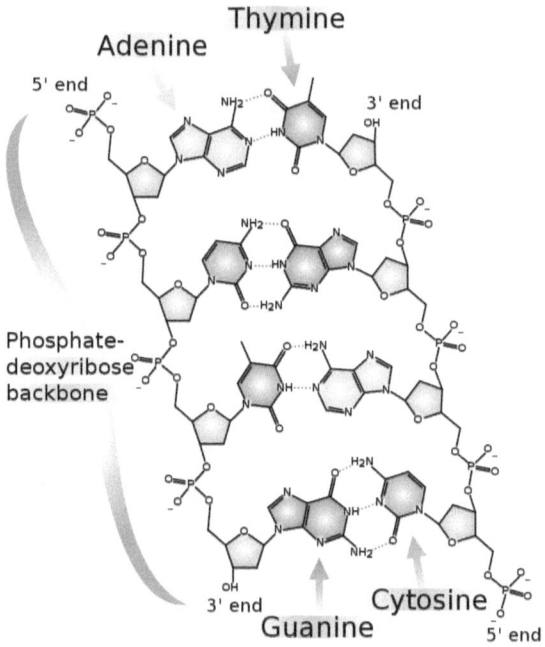

## DNA CEMICHICAL STRUCTURE

Specific genes are replicators of the same chemicals, with one difference—their biological units are very small. The gene functions continuously and stays functional by keeping its machine (body) working, but only if it can get the exact chemicals from food that it needs.

*A recent* Scientific American *article and other internet sources (under micro RNA) indicated that products of all plants following absorption in bloodstreams are in the form of micro RNA, which controls the output of by-products. This again confirms and substantiates that food needs to have the exact chemistry that was intended.*

*Until recently we had no idea how our biological body stays healthy. Evidence from these new articles indicates real food (all are biological with exact chemistry) if taken, prevent bad things from happening to the body, which we are seeing in increasing numbers).*

If there are no exact chemicals, the genes fall apart (gene degeneration) and cannot deliver the exact chemical parts necessary for repair. Genes can only stay alive and keep functioning correctly if they get the exact food chemistry they need to sustain themselves and, in turn, the entire body. If the genes do not receive the exact chemicals necessary, they go through a process called gene degeneration, and as a result, will not be able to maintain and make the exact chemicals they are supposed to.

There are many, many genes in the body. Each gene is responsible to do an exact manufacturing. If exact manufacturing is done, then our body does proper repair because it is able to do so. The body will then function properly and not scream for help with pain.

If proper repair is not done because of body malfunction because of improper food chemicals, slowly you will be afflicted with all sorts of diseases that have metabolic origins: *high blood pressure, stroke, a variety of arthritis (different kinds of joint problems, tendon problems, ligament problems), diabetes, and so on. Pain* could start at the beginning before any of the above starts, or it could occur in conjunction with any of the above. Pain with time will get worse.

*Let us see what happens if the body cannot find the exact proper chemical(s) with the exact chemistry from the original food,* which is no longer available. Then it has to use the chemical(s) closest to it. These chemicals, which do not have the proper exact chemistry, are incorporated into your tissue. Then, as a result, the body machine will break down. The breakdown presents as disease(s), which make you go to the doctor with pain or other signs and symptoms.

*To be precise, as result of proper food intake, and proper (with exact chemistry) RNA transcription, it prevents abnormal protein compounds' to be made. For example it prevents cancer formation.*

*The same goes for all disease that is happening to all mankind.*

Wait, there is more:

*What is really happening now?*

In 1968, when I was in college, my final exam was an article from the *New York Times* stating a scientist was claiming that from an intestinal tadpole cell, he made a new tadpole. We were required to explain the validity of this claim and why we thought that way, on the basis of our knowledge, experience, and training.

A visiting professor was teaching the course from Melbourne University, in Australia, who was involved in research in cloning, in hopes that future man could produce organs to save people from organ failure.

*Where Are We Now?*

During my orthopedic training, which was over twenty years ago, the incidence of diabetes was less than 5 percent. In the past twenty years, it has increased at an alarming rate. Now over 50 percent of the American population is diabetic, according to a PRI-MED meeting in December 2009, which I attended. According to different speakers the rate of diabetes in the low income Hispanic population is going up at an alarming rate. This is due to the rate of consumption of yellow corn in corn tortillas. The rate among low-income blacks is not much better, due to consumption of fast food and sodas (from my own observation( analysis of our own patients), and also Pri Med meetings) .

It was thought that diabetes is genetic (hereditary) in nature. However, I see many families where the children are diabetic but not their parents. What this means is that other factors are involved. It is true, however, that if your parents have diabetes, you will be affected sooner or later in your life. But something in our life is causing these accelerated changes.

We know that the liver plays a great role in body metabolic activities. We know the liver is the controlling factor and the factory to filter or metabolize all bad things that we eat and change them to not be harmful to the body. The liver also plays a great role in development of diabetes (every patient with hepatitis, or HIV that I have seen by age 55 has diabetes). We know diabetes is of two types. Type two diabetes is also called insulin-resistant diabetes. Insulin is responsible for guiding sugar and carbohydrates into your cells for their consumption and function. Two scenarios can be thought of: Either sugar is abnormal so that the body rejects it by producing resistance to its availability in the cell. Or there may be too much sugar so that not all of it can be metabolized, again producing the same results. The third scenario is that both scenarios are at work.

If sugar is normal but you are using too much, this does not fit into the equation of diabetes, because we have always had people who used too much, but they were not diabetic. If sugar and carbohydrates are normal, the body can metabolize them or store them. We have always had people who had bigger appetites than normal. However, we never before saw obesity in America such as we have been seeing for the past eighteen to twenty years. Maybe people would become overweight, but we did not see nearly as much obesity as we see now.

We do not see diabetes in people who are over eighty years old nearly as prevalently as in those under eighty. Older people have eaten the same food but were not exposed to the chemicals in food at a young age.

We all ate fast foods over the last eighty years. From the movie of Super Size, we learned that fast food is causing fatty livers. We are seeing (my own patients) more and more in liver ultrasounds that fatty livers are prevalent in people who consume fast food and corn tortillas (the common denominator is corn and corn products). This was also confirmed by *Life Extension* magazine.

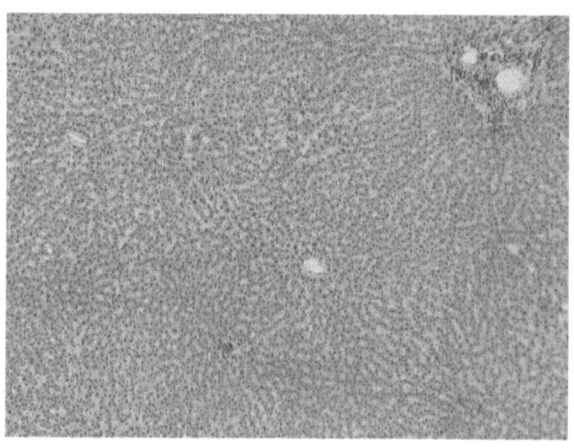

NORMAL LIVER HISTOLOGY- CELLS

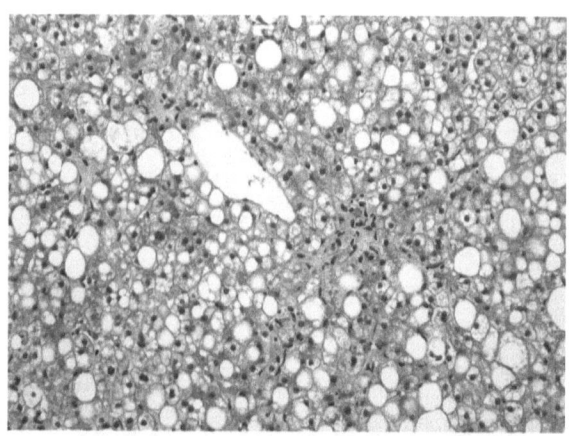

FATTY LIVER HISTOLOGY-CELLS

The movie *"Food, Inc."* showed us chickens that were being fed 100 percent genetically modified corn. Chicken in this movie were called "market ready" in six weeks time, in place of the normal six to twelve months' time Which are not fed yellow corn.

What does this mean? Because corn cannot be utilized and metabolized properly, the chickens are eating their food (corn), constantly, because they feel hungry all the time. It was being deposited in different body parts, including the liver and muscle mass under their skin. During these six weeks, almost 5 percent of the chickens died from organ failure. They were also prone to infections in spite of, being fed heavy doses of antibiotics.

This corn diet led to abnormal meat development in chickens and caused liver and renal failure. They also suffered lower resistance to infection and other diseases, seen also in humans today. This means that if the chickens are kept longer than six weeks, eventually all will die from the same problems.

There is evidence and reports from my patients who are suffering from chronic pain, when eating chicken and turkey meats; there is substantial increase in their pain. This was not the case before twenty-five years ago. The only things that have changed, is the ownership of hatcheries has gone from family control to the control of big fast-food companies, and their feed.

The chemistry of chicken meat and turkey meat has changed as a result of *genetically altered, genetically modified organisms* (GMO) feed. *A lot of food has changed directly, and some has changed indirectly.*

*The most common genetically modified food is corn, being used in cereal of all types, popcorn, as corn syrup in sodas, and in dog foods.* Dog foods have a large amount of corn and corn products in them. This explains the health problems developing in dogs in large number, such as diabetes, pancreatitis, and cancer.

*Genetically modified corn* was claimed to produce higher yield and not be affected by bugs, like all other GMO foods. Well, evidence documented by others indicates that more insecticide has to be used on the farms growing genetically modified corn. Since that has not worked, biotech companies have introduced self-contained insecticides in the chemistry of their products; called BT (Bacillus Thuringiensis, commonly found in soil (Under BT technology). It has been detected in the blood of pregnant mothers. The long-term consequences of it are yet unknown. But we know according to Internet sources honeybees were in proximity of GMO, cornfields with BT were dying in Poland. Then government of Poland voted against GMO food (under beekeepers win ban on GMO, s in Poland).

I am concerned if bugs do not eat a particular food or mold does not grow on it in a particular time span, what may be wrong with that food?

We have done studies on our own patients, comparing those who used GMO corn products versus those who used no GMO corn products. Those who consumed GMO corn products had a higher glycemic index than the non-GMO corn product consumers. As we stated previously, we were not seeing fatty livers in Hispanics over twenty-five years ago with the same food.

Our studies have shown that since there have been experimental farms of genetically altered wheat, they have contaminated and altered non-GMO farms through a very sophisticated systematic process called male killer genes by winds and flies. In our own patients, we see elevation of ANA (antinuclear antibody), increased TPO (thyroid peroxidase antibody), and thyroglobulin antibodies as a result.

For whatever reasons—which may not be explained entirely in this book—our body does not and will not like to use these foods; they are creating a lot of problems, as you are noticing in this book. Our body is not able to adapt to this *GMO food* due to certain changes that have been done to its gene structures and subsequently to its exact chemistry, which is different than that the original product.

In my observation, the majority of people develop obesity, diabetes, and other autoimmune disorders sooner or later—it's only a matter of time. A small percentage of the population, who control their calorie intake, will never gain weight; however, they develop the same diseases as obese people. There is one difference: the obese individual finds it easier to control his or her diabetes than the thin one, since by losing weight; we reduce the mass and therefore reduce the insulin requirements.

Do you know the latest tactic and funniest commercial on television? It states, "Your body does not recognize the difference between corn sugar and cane sugar." I have no idea where they got that from or what they are smoking. *This is total deception of the public regarding their health and right to know what is real and what is not.*

## The Effect of GMO in Our Food Chain

Fast forward to the present. This science of *genetic engineering* has advanced. A lot of biotech companies have jumped on the bandwagon to supposedly improve our food. *They can use the law of patenting to force all farmers to pay for seed and not be able to use their own seed from their own crops, which have been genetically modified.* As we all know, man has used nuts for thousands of years without one allergic response. There was no nut allergy until the nut was changed through genetic modification. Now, we have a large number of people who are deathly allergic to the GMO nuts.

Genetic modifications have been done to other products as well. Soy according to some was the first one to be altered (1966 soybean, corn, and later on, canola, rice and cotton seed oil= Under genetically modified food). From Internet source (form Organic Consumers site. More are coming, and being approved.

Two years ago, in an open letter, the government of Japan warned the US government that if their organic, non-genetically modified soy was processed on the same conveyer belt as the genetically modified soy, they were not going to buy their soy from the United States anymore. This should tell us the magnitude of problems they know about (from Organic Consumers Association site).

Currently wheat is causing considerable problems; a large number of people are developing ulcerative colitis, which is nothing more than an allergy of the gut or colon to this product. It also causes elevation of ANA (antinuclear antibodies, which are autoantibodies directed against the contents of the cell nucleus).

What does all this mean? It means that your own body cells, which are supposed to be present and functioning for a long time, are being destroyed slowly, but ultimately and surely.

## Inflammation and gene degeneration

To understand this better, let us see what an allergy is.

What is an allergy? An *allergy* to something means the body does not like it, so it rejects it, by attacking it through the immune system. Whatever the material or chemical or product is, regardless of its location, the body will attack it to get rid of it and destroy it because it detects it as a foreign substance that does not fit into the system or body or tissues.

Now let us see another aspect of this. If you eat a product, a small or minute amount of its components will go to the repair process and get incorporated into your body, as protein, carbohydrate, or fat. Through the RNA transcription process, it goes into the cells. Now your body police, which is your immune system, will identify the cell or tissue not to be normal, that is, as foreign. The immediate reaction of the body is to reject it. This rejection process is called an *allergic response.*

If this allergy occurs to tissue or an organ, it is called an *autoimmune reaction.* This means your body is attacking itself to destroy that part that does not have the exact genetic marker, code, chemistry, or structure that is normal. It is recognized or given identification that it is foreign, or enemy.

Let us see how our body defenses work against something that is not compatible with our system.

There are two systems in the body. One is an *antibody,* which is always present and can act immediately when it detects something bad or foreign in the body *and it has had previous experience with something similar.* It takes time to develop this (similar to vaccination we get). It can attack it and destroy it, by binding with it to neutralize the foreign substance before it harms the body.

The other system is *when the body has not seen the foreign object before.* First, it needs to find out what it is, to identify it by specific cells (B-lymphocytes) that are in the immune system. Then it tells the immune system to make antibodies. While making antibodies, it will call to action immediately other specific cells, which act like infantry or soldier cells (neutrophils, lymphocytes) to attack the foreign substance or tissue to clean up or destroy the abnormal tissues or cells or foreign material.

Sometimes, if the material or substance is too big, the immune system has cells (macrophages) to bite it into smaller pieces and then destroy it.

In the case of food, it becomes a bit more complicated. At the beginning, the food may not be recognized as GMO (abnormal chemistry). The GMO food will be identified at the last stage, when it is broken down into its basic component parts to be used by the body in the repair process.

When genes, the body repair factory, are forced to use the imitation chemicals or improper chemicals to do the repair process, defects start occurring. *The body, by attacking itself, by invading its own tissue, causes pain and inflammation.*

**What happens next, we all know, is very clear.**

What happens next is the very basis of the problem, called *autoimmune* disease. The abnormal chemical is used in the repair process, thus becoming a part of your muscle, a part of your thyroid, a part of your blood vessels, and a part of your joint.

Here, the problem starts again. The cells or tissues get a visit by the body police, the immune system. The immune system recognizes that the cells and the tissue have a problem. They do not have the exact chemistry components or chemicals; they were supposedly identified as normal, but they are not.

What happens now?

Your body attacks itself by its defenses, its armies; the immune system acts like Pac-Man (this is the process which causes inflammation and pain).

Now you have a very complicated situation in hand that our doctors are neither familiar with nor trained to handle.

Why?

The problem now is gene breakdown or degeneration. It can cause not only one problem, but also a combination of problems, because of the inability to do the proper repair process because the genes are malfunctioning due to lack of availability of proper chemicals or food components. Genes do more than one task at a time. The genes' preservation and also their functions are related to the exact chemistry of food and its availability to them.

So far you have noticed where the problem is. Because of lack of availability of exact food chemistry when incorporated into the body, the next sequence is that the body has to attack itself for preservation, because it now has identified an enemy; this is called an *autoimmune disorder*. *Autoimmune disorders develop if genes were not able to preserve their integrity by making the correct chemicals (protein) and not break down. You would think that when non-GMO food is given to these patients, it should correct the problems. But this does not happen. These patients or people feel better with non-GMO food, but if the situation is not corrected very early and damage is done to their gene sections, they still need-modified treatment.*

## Autoimmune Disorders

Let us see what are possible causes of the above complaints.

The above problems are all related to a category of diseases called *autoimmune disorders*. This is nothing except a complex of allergy-related conditions with grave lifetime consequences.

They are conditions in which your body attacks your own body and destroys your body in one form or the other for the reasons explained above. The affected organ gets a visit from the body police, the immune system. The body police attacks the affected organ and presents itself as inflammation, which is followed by pain in the corresponding area, which most of the time starts in a muscle group (shoulder muscles, back muscles, neck muscles, etc.). The inflammation starts in one area of the body and then goes to a different area of body muscle groups. The start and spreading of inflammation has to do with the workload, particular body parts, and blood supply to the muscle groups and facial areas. This explains the pain pattern. Soon stiffness will follow, which is documented in every rheumatology book and related subjects.

What are some common examples of autoimmune disorders?

*Rheumatoid arthritis:* Usually presents with symmetrical (both right and left sides) joint swelling, pain, and stiffness. This worsens over several weeks. There are also patients who develop the late manifestation, with ulna drift (fingers tilt toward the outside) and tendonitis in the wrist early rather than swelling of the joint and pain.

*Psoriatic arthritis:* Early symptoms are pain in the extremity and not necessarily in the joint (like tennis elbow or hip tendonitis). The joint later becomes inflamed and also has stiffness. All patients have psoriatic skin changes (silvery looking discoloration) at the back of the elbows. Eventually most will develop diabetes too.

*Lupus:* Presents with fatigue, malaise, and joint pain with stiffness. Fever and node swelling are present. A butterfly rash on the face is present in 50 percent of patients.

*Hashimoto's thyroiditis: inflammation of thyroid gland, which causes eventually loss of thyroid function or decreases production of thyroid hormone.*

*Sjogren's syndrome:* Develops very slowly. Manifests as dry eye and mouth. Eyes become itchy and feel like there is sand in them.

*Mixed autoimmune disorder:* Fatigue, malaise, joint pain, stiffness, or renal problem. Presentation is a mixed bag, as the name implies.

*Polyarthropathy:* Multiple joints and muscle groups are involved; starts in one place and progresses to other joints relatively quickly with stiffness.

*Diabetes:* The earliest sign could be lack of sleep. As time goes on, there is joint manifestation. Pain occurs in different joints, most commonly the shoulders and knees. The rest of the symptoms related to diabetes come later and not as initial problems.

*Polymyalgia rheumatic and giant cell arteritis:* Presents with aching, morning stiffness in the shoulder and hip. Fatigue and malaise also are present.

*Fibromyalgia:* Presents with tissue pain, skin becomes very sensitive to touch sensation changes sleep disturbance and stiffness. Skin nerve ending becomes very sensitive to touch. Also their muscles become very sensitive. So far, we have found it to be a combination of insulin resistance (with normal sugar and HBA1C) and polyarthropathy.

*Complex regional pain syndrome:* Usually follows a simple trauma, or after surgery due to an injury. The affected part becomes very sensitive and painful to even touch and is very sensitive to cold exposure. Patients also have stiffness and joint pain.

*Ulcerative colitis and inflammatory bowel disease:* Presents with abdominal pain, gas, and persistent diarrhea. Patients also have joint pain and stiffness.

*Gout:* Usual presentation is joint swelling, pain, and warmth in affected part. Usually seen in the foot as plantar fasciitis and ankle (also knee and hip), and not so much in the big toe anymore.

Fifty to seventy-five percent of rheumatoid arthritis patients also suffer from thyroid problems and diabetes. Similarly, twenty-five to thirty percent of patients with thyroid problems and diabetes also suffer from rheumatoid arthritis. A large number also suffer from gout.

Another condition people suffer from is *unexplained hip pain*. These people often have an MRI and then are diagnosed with ligament problems. Arthroscopic surgery follows, which does nothing for them at all. Soon they develop arthritis, with a lot of pain, and need total hip replacement at a very early age. Sometimes people are wrongfully diagnosed with osteomyelitis. They are even subjected to open hip surgery to look into the joint to drain suspected pus, which is not there.

*What are the long-term consequences of the improper treatment of all the above conditions?*

In the case of diabetes:

- Cataracts will develop, resulting in optic neuropathy and blindness.
- Over time, memory problems and loss will occur.
- Neck and upper back pain starts involving the shoulders.
- There is also arm pain, and numbness in the hands.
- There may be mid-back pain.
- Some develop abdominal pain.
- Some develop an ovarian cyst and abdominal pain.

- The majority of patients have lower back pain.
- Most females have sacral pain, and the elderly have incontinence of urine.
- In men, it causes a prostate problem.
- The leg may become painful; heel pain, ankle pain, and foot pain may start, and with time will get worse.

Some develop wound-healing problems and do not respond to any treatment; then They need to have Hyper-Baric chamber, extensive wound treatment, and plastic flap surgery to close the wound. Later they lose circulation in the lower leg, causing gangrene, followed by amputation.

Another serious problem happening more and more frequently in our society is super infection in the form of hospital-acquired infections or none hospital form.

Also, people are becoming more and more prone to infections because of diminished immune systems and lack of proper blood flow to the tissues.

*The common denominator of all of the above autoimmune disorders is micro capillary vasculitis and more.*

## What is capillary vasculitis?

Capillary Vasculitis is the inflammation of the lining of blood vessels. If large vessels are involved, inflammation of the inner lining will narrow the lumen, but not impede the blood flow.

When small blood vessels, called arterioles, are affected by inflammation, it causes serious problems. These arterioles are so tiny in diameter that only one small red cell, a few microns in size, can pass through at a time. So when arterioles start becoming inflamed, it impedes (obstructs, prevents, or slows down) the flow of blood to the tissue. When blood vessels are affected (inflamed) due to this condition, the blood flow interference can be documented by a three-phase bone scan. The blood pressure slowly goes up in order to compensate for the slowdown of blood flow to the tissues. Slowly this problem becomes worse and worse with time. Sometimes you are placed on multiple blood pressure medications, but still your blood pressure is not under control.

If your tissues, which make up your entire body (think skin, tendons, joints, cartilage, muscles, and organs), do not receive enough blood and nutrients on time, then they experience myriad unwanted effects:

- The *skin* gets dry, develops hyper pigmentation initially, and over time becomes darker and darker in color. The surface of the skin loses hair.

- *Tendons* develop tendonitis. (Tendons have a very limited blood supply.) Nutrients flow to the tendons from the tendon sheet and its secretions. Lack of blood flow causes inflammation of the tendon initially, and then tendonapathy (which is degeneration of the core substance of the tendon) will develop.
  If you are experiencing foot pain in the bottom of your foot and have difficulty walking, you are told you have plantar-fasciitis. If you have shoulder pain and your rotator cuff is inflamed, you are told you have impingement and you need surgery. Unless the disease is brought under control, surgery will not help you. Eventually, your rotator cuff will tear and get disrupted. If knee pain occurs, then you are told you need surgery. Again, that will not help you. When you develop hip pain, you are told you need an MRI, and then hip surgery, starting with arthroscopy.

- *Joints (cartilage)* do not have enough blood supply to receive their nutrients, so arthritis begins to set in. Joints obtain nutrients from secretions that come from the membrane, called a synovial membrane, inside the joint. When the disease process occurs, this membrane slowly loses the ability to secret the proper synovial fluid (with the proper chemical structure) for nutrition of the cartilage. Under normal circumstances, after this fluid is secreted, it does not directly flow to the cartilage cells. It gets to the cells by what is called compression and diffusion. That means, when you move your joints by the activities of daily living, this fluid is pushed into the cells. This is the normal way nutrients get into the cells of cartilage.

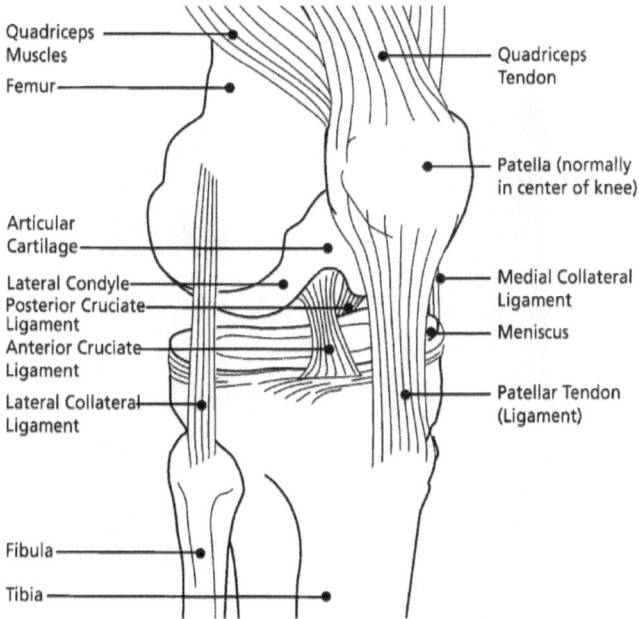

**KNEE ANATOMY**

John Kayvanfar, MD

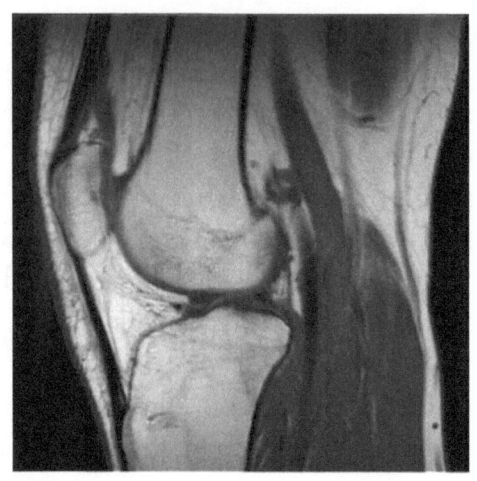

## KNEE ANATOMY ON MAGNETIC RESONANCE IMMIGING

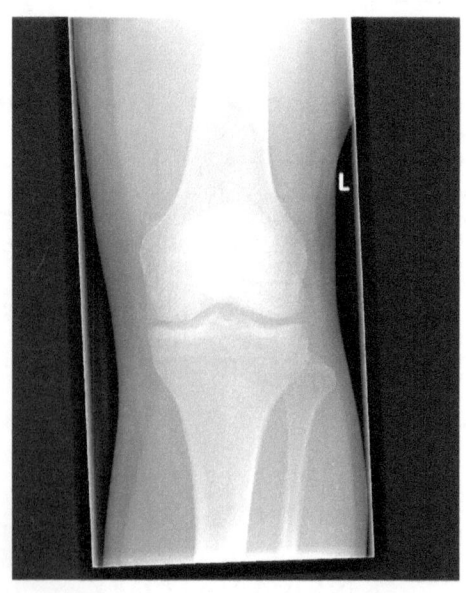

## X-RAY OF NORMAL KNEE

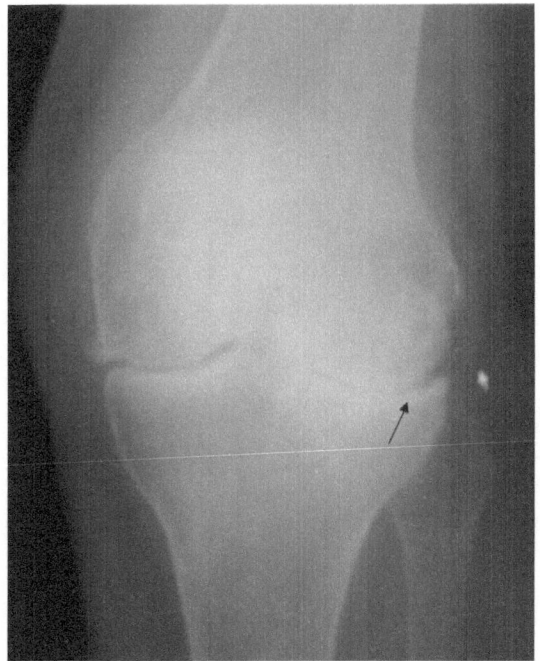

## X-RAY OF KNEE WITH ARTHRITIS

The first stage is that the synovial tissue will look pale; with time, it will develop hypertrophy to compensate for the lack of secretions or the improper chemical structure, and it will develop Villi type inflammation, which is abnormal (this membrane is normally red). Most of the time, other changes occur. Now the synovial membrane is unable to deliver the proper form of nutrients to the joint cells. Once this process starts, the joint cartilage starts developing degeneration, called chondromalacia, and bony spurs on the margin of the joints. This time the radiologist reads the changes as degenerative joint disease. Actually, you are developing arthropathy, which is degeneration of the cartilage, or arthritis.

Sooner or later, you are sent to an orthopedist. He orders X-rays and an MRI. Radiologists and regular orthopedists do not know the significance of a cyst that may develop below the joint margin. The cyst that develops signifies an autoimmune disorder, not degenerative joint disease.

The knee meniscus becomes worn and fragile with time, and will tear apart under slight load. The meniscus is a C-shaped cartilage in the knee. The meniscus receives its nutrients on the outer surface directly from the blood supply. The periphery of the meniscus is thicker. The inner surface and margin is thinner and receives nutrients from the synovial fluid that is secreted into the knee. Once an autoimmune disorder happens or diabetes, this important tissue in the knee becomes weak and brittle, instead of being like rubber and hard. First, the meniscus becomes fragile in the center, and later on it develops an inter substance degeneration. As a result, it tears apart, called a horizontal clevelege-tear. The same goes for an ACL (anterior cruciate ligament) tear with trivial or slight trauma. Now you need ACL reconstruction or surgery. Normally ACL tears with a severe and forceful force to the knee. Now you are told you need arthroscopic surgery.

Once you develop advanced chondromalacia, or arthritis, you are told you have bad joint arthritis and now you need total joint replacement.

- *Muscles* become painful and tender too. You try to do more and more exercise, but nothing works on it. Then you are sent to pain management. Now you are going to get some sort of pain medication or combinations, in the form of different classes of pain medication. Then your pains are going to get stronger as time goes on. Then you will receive more and stronger medications.

- Your *heart* may become irritable and slowly develop arrhythmia. Now you are to see a cardiologist. Next come EKG or ECG tests. If you have arrhythmia, you definitely need some medicine, because if you do not get help or medicine, you could die.

- The *lung* develops fibrosis in a later stage. Now you may need a sleep study and medicine or a gadget to better sleep.

- As a result of GMO food, the *liver* will accumulate fat and develop a fatty liver. This condition reduces its capacity to function.

- Your *brain* initially develops fatigue, and you slowly become forgetful. You may not be able to sleep. You may also develop sleep apnea. Sometimes you develop uncontrolled movement of the leg(s) associated with pain at night. Now you have restless or crazy leg syndrome. Now you definitely need proper medication to bring it under control so you can sleep.

- *Bones* are affected, too, and develop osteoporosis. Now you receive osteoporosis medication, which is not going to work completely if you do not get magnesium, calcium, and vitamin D in proper proportions. After you receive medication for osteoporosis only, you may feel better temporarily or not at all. Then you are back to square one. This picture goes on for a while, but you are getting worse, and it is only a matter of time before your bones start collapsing, getting fragile and breaking with minimal trauma.

*Glands* are also being affected and become involved slowly by becoming weaker in their function.

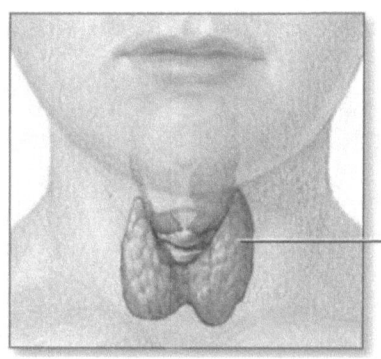

Glande thyroïde

# PLACE AND SHAPE OF THYROID GLAND IN THE BODY

## Thyroid system

Hypothalamus

Anterior pituitary gland

Thyrotropin-releasing hormone (TRH)

Negative feedback

Thyroid-stimulating hormone (TSH)

Thyroid gland

**Thyroid hormones (T3 and T4)**

**Increased metabolism**
Growth and development
Increased catecholamine effect

# RELATIONSHIP OF THROID GLAND AND PETUITARY GLAND IN THE BODY

A lot of people are subjected to a lot of unnecessary surgeries.

So, you see, the true cause of the problems is missed entirely.

Why? Because the above course of treatment is the standard of care at the present time.

# Chapter Three

## Why Treatments Are Not Working

### The Problems with Deduction

A combination of diseases means complicated testing and deduction. When you are affected by different disease combinations together, that needs to be recognized simultaneously and needs to be corrected and treated; otherwise, it causes multiple problems, and your body is going to continue experiencing and presenting the problem(s) with pain.

Unfortunately, medicine is too specialized. This means you see the primary care, family practice, general practice, or internal medicine doctor first.

First, the doctor must recognize there are multiple problems. Then he needs to refer you to the correct specialist on time. This happens only rarely. As a result, you end up with pain management, which is the wrong place to be.

Let us assume your primary care physician is great and a very aware individual. He will see you and order tests on the basis of his education and knowledge.

The blood tests he orders consist of CBC (complete blood count), differential (measures number of WBC, or white blood cells = between 4000.0 to 11000.0; differential (percentage of different cells under normal circumstances) needs to be, neutrophils around 68%, lymphocytes also around 26%, and mono less than 5%), TSH (needs to be below 2.0 in 99 percent of population), LFT (test function of liver and any stress or abnormality; lab values are correct), BUN (blood urea nitrogen/ waste product from body = the lower the number the better), creatinine (which measures the rate of glomerular filtration of kidney = the lower the number the better), and fasting blood sugar (needs to be below 90, and not 100 or any other number).

When you go for the next visit or you're called on the phone, you are told the results are normal. Then you ask, "If the results are normal, how come I do not feel normal?" When you pose this question to your doctor, he states he does not know. He is right—because he looks at your lab data with reference to the normal range. Every lab test comes with reference results, what is normal and what is not normal. The problem is that the references vary from one lab to the next. The references are not standardized throughout the United States, and some references date from the World War II era. Some of these references are not normal anymore. For instance, the TSH result needs to be between 0.3 and 2.0 to be normal. However, labs today give you 0.3 to 4.5 or even 5.5 as normal.

Fasting blood sugar is a very unreliable test, because its value depends on what you ate and when you ate the night before. If you ate at 6:00 p.m. or at 9:00 p.m., of course your results would be different.

Cell count can be looked at in different ways. If your red cells are within normal limits but at the lower limits of normal, this could mean relative anemia, which could represent a disease or rheumatoid condition.

White cells can also be looked at in different ways. The total count could be within normal limits. However, there are different types of WBC (white blood cells), and each needs to be at a specific number and percentage. Changes in the percentage of each could represent a disease process.

## Health Entities' Roles

The tests that are not done are significant and are called specialized tests, but your primary care physician can order them.

Those HMOs (health maintenance organizations) that do everything internally and do not accept any outside orders or prescriptions are the worst in the system. Even if you could afford to go and see an outside doctor and he recommended what you need, those HMOs would not order the proper blood tests or give you the needed medicine. They always tell you that you do not need the tests. *Do you know why?* Once the test is run, the result always demonstrates there is something wrong that needs to be treated—but guess what! Once they find something is wrong and you need a referral to some sort of specialist, it costs money to treat you.

You need to ask your doctor, "If I do not need treatment, then why do I have pain and suffering?" (I must mention that not all doctors within HMOs are closed-minded).

Do you know what is the most pathetic statement I have ever heard from some of my patients? That the HMO doctor has told them, "You do not need the test" or "We know better than outside doctors."

Some other HMO's may want to save money to increase their margin of profit, make excuses not to do your tests, because it is less expensive to give you pain pills, than actually find the cause of your problems and treat you. However now you know the long-term consequences, of not being treated properly.

The tests you need to have now are to help to diagnose and pinpoint the problem(s) you have now; it is not simply enough to order the most common tests. In my opinion, *Any problem going on now in the United States and seen in regular medical offices that have to deal with pain without a history of trauma most are autoimmune in nature.*

Senior health plans are also becoming picky. If the doctor's office forgets to write the diagnosis on the labs, the insurance does not cover the cost of the test. Then the seniors end up being billed for the tests, ordering them to pay with money they do not have.

## Normal Lab Values Are Standardized—Or Accurate

The consequence of standard lab values allowing higher numbers is the development of cardiovascular problems. We all know the long-term consequences and astronomical costs associated with cardiovascular problems. The purpose of testing must be to control and normalize the patients' physiology to bring their long-term risk factors as close as possible to those of normal people. The numbers should not and must not be decided by just a collection of data from people and then coming up with some mathematical number from a bell-shape curve that has nothing to do with normal physiology.

The numbers need to be changed on the basis of normal physiology of normal and controlled subjects from all around the world, especially people from nations with the least number of health problems. Following is a list of suggested values:

TSH = between 0.3 and 2.0

HBA1c = must be less than 5.7 and not 5.7. The lower the better, depending on the problem and ethnicity. (There are people with normal HBA1c of 4.1, and there are people who are diabetic with HBA1c of 5.5.)

Uric acid = needs to be less than 6.0 and not just 6.0. If 6.0 were normal, they would not be coming to see a doctor.

Fasting blood sugar = can be used for reference and to monitor the response of patients. Needs to be below 90.0.

This way we would not have to pay expensive taxpayer money for wound healing. Normal people do not have any wound healing problems. The purpose of any treatment must be to imitate/mimic the physiology of normal people for patients who are suffering from all these conditions including wound-healing patients. In our own practice all the wounds, /diabetic ulcers heal without all these extra ordinary measure/treatments (oxygen, hyper baric chambers, different topical applications ("your body shall heal"), if you make the physiology normal.

We must look at the whole picture and decide on treatment. Some patients do need treatment, but some do not. There are patients with HBA1c of 6.1 who are not diabetic yet, so they do not need treatment.

## Misleading Information Yields Misleading Treatments, Which Do Not Work

If you only look at lab result numbers without looking at signs and symptoms, you are getting misleading information. Such results may not show the inflammatory marker characteristic of autoimmune disorders. The hallmark of autoimmune disorders is stiffness, regardless of lab numbers.

If you are very, very slowly and gradually developing stiffness in the morning, as time goes on, again very slowly, you will get worse. Besides, pain starts in one place and then expands to other places.

When you go to see your doctor, you complain only about pain in the most painful place in your body. So your doctor concentrates only on one place in your body. Usually you are having problems in more than one area of the body. Let us assume the pain is in your lower back, neck, shoulder, knee, or ankle, and the foot is the main problem. You get an X-ray of that particular part. You are prescribed anti-inflammatory medications (Naprosyn / Anaprox, Motrin / ibuprophen) and pain medication. You take the prescriptions for a while, and you do not get better. Now your doctor may consider also prescribing physical therapy for you or sending you to an orthopedist.

When your orthopedist sees you at your appointment, you complain again of the most painful area in your body. Your orthopedist either examines that area, or if you are lucky, may examine that extremity and related parts. After evaluation, the orthopedist orders another X-ray and changes your anti-inflammatory medication, or you may get an order for an MRI of the part. Now you have the X-ray and MRI. On reading the results, you are given a diagnosis as follows:

If you are an adult and you have complained of neck pain, you probably have some arthritis in your neck. You are told you have osteoarthritis in your neck. The orthopedist offers you stronger pain medication and another class of anti-inflammatory medicine. Either you feel somewhat better or not. If you feel better, that may continue indefinitely. If you do not feel better, they recommend you to have pain management (Lyrica/Neurontin or narcotics) or surgery.

If you have shoulder pain, the same recommendations are followed: anti-inflammatory medicine, pain medication, X-rays, and finally an MRI and physical therapy. The MRI shows you have inflammation, and it is read as impingement. When you do not respond to therapy, you may be recommended to have surgery.

If the pain is in your hand and you have pain and numbness, you are diagnosed with carpal tunnel syndrome. Again, you are given anti-inflammatory medications and may receive a steroid shot. Then when the problem does not go away, it is suggested you have electromyography (EMG), a nerve conduction study (NCV) for carpal tunnel syndrome, and surgery for your problem.

If the body part experiencing pain happens to be your back, the same treatment plan is followed as your neck: first, anti-inflammatory medicine and pain medicine, and then an X-ray. After that comes a consultation with an orthopedist. Then comes the MRI, followed by therapy.

If the MRI shows arthritis and possibly some bulging discs and you are not responding to treatment, then surgery is recommended. You may also get a recommendation for epidural injections.

A small percentage of the population feels chest pain, and all experience problems with sleeping (which can be the earliest sign of Diabetes). Pleurisy or Pericarditis, can be representation of rheumatoid condition. A considerable number of people experience allergy and asthma. A large number of people present with dry eye. All of them, need proper treatment.

I have great advice for everyone: *If your doctor makes a diagnosis for you and treats you with medicine or surgery for the condition, you do not respond, do not get better, the wrong diagnosis was given to you. Also, there may be other problems in the equation, which are being missed.*

# Chapter Four

## How You Can Take Control Of Your Health

### Making Sure Your Doctor Assesses the "Whole Picture"

When the above conditions are happening to people, what are adults told to do? A lot of people who are having aches and severe pain, stiffness, and lack of sleep or insomnia are told, "You are just getting old." I have news for you: I know of ninety-three-year-olds who have no problems.

*All* such problems are related to autoimmune disorders (metabolic problems also need to be put into this category). Unfortunately, a good number of these patients do not present with conventional blood changes initially, and therefore they do not receive the proper treatment. The hallmark symptom of all autoimmune disorders is morning stiffness, regardless of lab test results. The earliest symptom of diabetes, contrary to what is stated in books, is lack of sleep at night, again regardless of lab values. (If there are abnormal lipid/cholesterol values, in the majority of cases, this is the beginning of insulin resistance.)

To get a proper diagnosis, first, one needs to get a proper and complete history (full review of systems) and then undergo a full physical examination. The physical examination must be thorough, starting from the outside to inside and from top (the head) to toe.

Taking a good and complete history takes time. And you, being an informed consumer, can choose your doctor accordingly. Similar problems do not all have the same solutions.

Doctors have been paid less and less for the last twenty-five years, while medicine has become more complicated. And the cost of everything, including an office practice, has gone up considerably. In Canada last year, they doubled the pay to physicians for offices and consultation.

The bottom line is that doctors are not being paid a fair share of collected insurance premiums.

Who ends up at the short end of the stick? All of us, who sooner or later become patient and need medical care; Even though you may have a lot of money, since the system is set up the way it is, it will not bring your health back properly.

As one learns the basics in medical school, treatment starts with a good and complete history by the doctor. In order to get a good history, the doctor needs to take a thorough muscular skeletal history from head to toe, not just of a part of the body, which is typical for all subspecialties. Most patients who go to see doctors usually complain of the most severe pain, but it is the doctor who should question the patients thoroughly to get to the bottom of the problems.

As is stated in medical school, a history is more than 70 percent of the diagnosis.

Usually patients have problems in one or more areas and go to a doctor to seek medical attention for the most severe problem. If asked carefully about other parts of the body, each individual will agree that he or she has pains in other parts of the body. All have difficulty sleeping, and all are stiff in the morning for a short time or longer.

The physical examination should be thorough from head to toe. Every muscle group, tendon, and joint in the body should be examined and documented.

Then come the lab orders. You need to request that your doctor order a complete blood test as designated below.

Lab tests to order:

CBC, Differential, and ESR

ANA, RF, and CRP = all quantitatively

HgA1c

Uric Acid

BUN, Creatinine, and GFR

LFT

TSH, Thyroid Peroxidase, and Thyroglobulin

DS DNA

ASO titer

Maybe consider a complete lupus panel

Autoimmune diseases are caused by a combination of direct lymphocyte infiltrations and autoantibody response.

## Treatment

Next comes the more complicated part of the treatment, which are the medications. This is *the real art*. Why is this the real art? Because in medicine, two and two is not always four, even though in math it is always four.

Because each body is slightly different from each other, the status of organ systems could vary. If one has a bad kidney, he or she cannot receive certain medications that might damage the kidney further, and close monitoring must be done on the kidney. This means urine tests and blood tests need to be ordered very frequently, at least every three months. If the tests are not done in short intervals, more kidney damage will occur, and the patient ends up needing continuous renal dialysis. At that point it costs the system more money to keep you around. You may need a kidney or renal transplant.

Last point, one cannot rely solely on the blood test. We have been developing new blood tests all the time, to detect new conditions, but still are short for proper documentation and evidence that a particular diagnosis exists. Again complete symptoms and signs (complete history and physical exam) is the most important part of the evaluation for treatment. You do not need necessarily to have positive blood test to be treated properly for your condition.

## Finding Out Whether Your Food Is Safe

Now you are beginning to understand what is happening to all of us and why.

Our healthy and prosperous existence depends on what we eat. Proper food with proper chemistry is the answer. Just like your car depends on good gas and service, your body is even more precise in what it needs and uses. Let us see how and what food gives to us.

The Food and Drug Administration (FDA) approves what food and drugs can be sold. Just like cigarettes, whose manufacturers claimed *their products* to be harmless, food is handled the same way by the FDA. Finally cigarette labels were changed. The big companies tell the EPA and FDA their products are safe to eat. The FDA never requires multicenter studies in animals that have eaten GMO foods to see if they are safe or not. There are studies done at a lot of places, including our own universities in this country that confirm the problems with GMO.

The biotech companies claim that their food is safe, but it is not. I can state this not only because of my experience with my patients, but also because of tons of information on the Internet. For example, Ron Fried reported on Tuesday, November 28, 2000, that Doctor John Hagelin presented a paper to the Environmental Protection Agency. This presentation indicated the allergenic effect of Star Link corn on human health. Star Link corn was found to be contaminated by GMO corn that had not been approved by the FDA/EPA for human consumption.

What to eat and not to eat in short: *For now, my advice for all of us is to avoid foods that are harmful and consume more foods that still may be not so harmful.* Here are some specific guidelines:

- Buy as much as you can organic from trusted sources since, there are no real published guidelines from the Department of Agriculture relating to GMO.
- Avoid all wheat, corn, some of the white rice, and most of soy products. This includes fast foods and most cereals.
- Avoid all sodas.
- Do not buy fruits and vegetables that are exactly the same size and shape; their exact same size and shape shows they are cloned or GMO.

- Buy fruits and vegetables that used to have seeds and still have the same amount of seeds.

- Eat fruits, rather than juice. Fruits are absorbed over a two-hour period, whereas fruit juice is absorbed within a few minutes, which requires a sudden discharge of insulin, which is a stress to the pancreas.

- It is more important to have good fat and not so much protein. (The majority of protein products are soy based or contain GMOs, which in general are harmful to kidneys and damage the system.) Our brain and neurological systems are made from fat. All our hormones are made from fat. We need good fats and oils, such as olive oil and sesame oil. Avocado is great for your body. All raw nuts are good to eat.

- A combination of good whole milk products and no-salt butter (with vitamin K2) is great to avoid osteoporosis.

- Breakfast must be your most important meal of the day. I recommend cheese, eggs, and butter from whole milk and not low fat dairy. Most low-fat dairy consists of bad fat (low-density fat) because when it is centrifuged to convert to low fat, the first fat to go out is the good fat, HDL.

- The best choice of bread at the present time is Ezekiel, because so far it is made of non-GMO products and contains a lot of protein, so you need less meat to eat.

*Make sure you buy true organic.* (I still have no idea how *organic* is defined by the FDA and Department of Agriculture and how it is defined by each state.) *You need to make sure your food is free of all insecticides and so forth and that it is not GMO (genetically engineered food).* We know what products are changed and are not what God gave us (soy, white rice, rye, barley, wheat, corn, tomato, cucumber, watermelon, cantaloupe, yum, sweet potato, and potato). Try to buy from your local organic farmers' market. Such markets have sponsors, mostly are informed about these things.

The Department of Agriculture needs to define for the people what is Organic. It must not bring the standard down to benefit some large companies at the expense of public health. True organic must be without the use of any insecticide and not be GMO.

Drugs go through rigorous FDA requirements for safety reasons. Drugs are tested in animals and volunteers for at least five years, culminating the fifteen years of study before they are released on the market. The same should apply to GMO foods, which are in reality a new chemical for human and animal use. Why do we care about what animals (including cows, sheep, goats, poultry, and fish) eat? Because we humans consume animal products that could in turn affect us.

## *Do You Know What* Kosher *Means?*

*Kosher* is a Hebrew word for healthy food. It means healthy by all means. That means no chemicals of any types (no insecticides, no pesticides, no hormones, no antibiotics of any type). According to kosher laws, if an animal is limp, it is not supposed to be used for food. After sacrificing the animal, two major organs must be free of diseases. One is the lung, which is exposed to environmental factors in the air; and the second is the liver, which filters the absorbed material from the gut before it gets to the rest of the body. Unfortunately this law is no longer in practice in the real setting and practice even for kosher meats. If it were, most of the meat that is being used would not be eligible for pass by kosher laws. The problem is the new Rabbi's do not check every liver and if they do, forget how the real liver looks and feels like. Because of the volume being too much or it is impractical to check every animal thoroughly.

If GMO food is causing autoimmune disorders, fatty livers, and lung fibrosis, do you think it is kosher to eat them? Either the animals are not checked thoroughly or the animals are killed before organ failure occurs, which would demonstrate the magnitude of the problem GMO food created in the organs.

If you are a mother, you are told not to take a lot of things—no coffee, no medications of any type, for example. What do you think that means? It means such things are harmful to the baby; this is what medical doctors say to pregnant women. If the substances are harmful to the baby, do you think they are not harmful to the mothers? If they are harmful to a mother, wouldn't they be harmful to a father? Don't you think they'd be harmful to the rest of us? You see how the medical community contradicts themselves.

Come on; think a little.

You and me and the rest of us are being played with. They always manage to find someone who does not have enough scientific background to comment that the GMO foods have no problems. This is the way they fooled the Marlboro Man to advertise about cigarettes, which were not safe. Finally he died from the severe consequences.

To paraphrase the final words of the Marlboro Man: "If I were aware of the consequences of my smoking and advertising, I wouldn't have done the advertising, even if I were offered all of the gold from the planet earth."(Marlboro Man's dying words Internet).

*Let us see what happens to those millions who use these foods.*

Once the standard treatment fails, you are pushed onto another specialty called pain management. These specialists are trained to only deal with chronic pain. So they give you different pain medications to keep you comfortable. The medications consist of different types of pain relievers that work in different parts of the body to block the pain from being experienced by your brain. They may also add a prescription for antidepressant medication at very high doses. But the medications do not stop the cause of pain because your body is being eaten piece by piece by your own immune system, like Pac-Man is eating products.

Let's see what the consequences are of using those medications. They consume all the enzymes that are needed for the body to repair itself. These enzymes are no longer available to do their necessary job of being involved in the repair process. This means your body can no longer make the products or chemicals needed to do a good repair job. As a consequence of the failure to stop the cause of pain, and due to the ongoing pain, your life is miserable. You cannot function properly and cannot do your daily activities properly. Because of chronic pain and organ damage, your life will be shorter, and eventually disability will occur.

## Let us see what the consequences are for future generations and how we all can help.

Diseases that are transferred from one generation to the next, such as diabetes, usually occur in the next generation at a younger age. What does this mean? It means that diseases are causing disability to appear in a younger age group with each subsequent generation.

Diabetes is one of the diseases that occur as a result of an autoimmune disorder. We always hear that if you are diabetic, your children will be diabetic. Also, if you have rheumatoid arthritis, your children will be affected. This transfer is called a genetic or hereditary transfer.

As I mentioned above, at the present time, 50 percent of Americans are diabetic according to a report at a Pri-Med meeting (continuous educational meeting for doctors) that I attended in December 2009. At this conference, it was mentioned that the rate of diabetes within the low income groups of Hispanic and black populations was going through the roof due to their pattern of food consumption. Do you think this is going to get better? It would be a joke if anyone told you it would. You can imagine the long-term consequences of autoimmune disorders and disability at a younger age on the workforce of this nation in the future.

The next question is how we can help people who currently have these diseases and those who will be developing them in the future. Those who are currently being affected need to be evaluated thoroughly for all possible combinations of diseases in order to do the proper treatment. Insurance companies that refuse to pay for the tests you need, without having enough knowledge of the situation, make it very difficult to practice real medicine.

Just like any other situation, if something is causing a problem, the cause needs to be removed. People need to be informed of what the bad foods are. The major GMO foods are corn, soy, white rice, potato, sugar beats, zucchini, and Alfa Alfa (officially) sweet potato, yam, rye, and barley (none officially/experimental), and all related products. Some of the same foods are being fed to animals, poultry, and farm-raised fish. In turn, we use their meat for human consumption. Our experience and evidence on the Internet show that such products are not healthy for consumption.

The problem is that all autoimmune disorders also affect blood vessels. Therefore, CRP/ C-reactive protein (which could indicate inflammation from the blood vessels) needs to be taken care of and be brought down by all possible means. If not, patients are at risk of bone necrosis, heart trouble, osteoporosis, stroke, arthritis, and more.

What organs remain safe in the body? There is really no organ that remains safe in the body.

We see a lot more people with chronic pain than previously, who also have different presentations of their symptoms.

For example, we see a lot more people who have elevated ANA antibody. What does that mean? It means your rate of actual cells being destroyed by your body has gone up. Most people with elevated ANA present with a lot of aches and pains in the body. So far we have seen this to be mostly related to *genetically modified products and related products, such as beer and liquors.*

We may have had cirrhosis in the past from alcohol consumption. However, we did not notice any fatty liver or autoimmune disorders from alcoholic drinks before.

*As a result of modification of our practice,* our patients are being treated with accurate history taking, examination of the entire body, and proper blood tests, followed by proper diet and medication. With the above treatment, there has been very little need for back surgeries, arthroscopic surgeries, total joint replacement, or carpal tunnel surgeries compared to my previous standard of practice.

## Spreading the Word

Use of chemical insecticides and herbicides needs to stop, and we need to find natural products like tobacco water or some other ways to deal with this issue. An agriculture engineer told me once that *tobacco* soaked in water is the most powerful natural insecticide.

Companies that are in the business of selling food should not be in the business of production of meat and vegetables too.

There must be guidelines for what can go into our food when it is sold.

There must be guidelines and criteria for what birds and animals can be killed as food in our country.

Companies that produce seeds cannot be in charge of food production, too, in the same way that a drug is not tested by pharmaceutical companies, but by independent doctors and their patients.

Genetically modified food needs to stop being produced and sold in our country until there is proof and data about its safety. Food and its chemistry is a very complex issue; it is not simple. The issue is not just bugs attacking the food, and let's does something to produce more food for the population; the most important issue must be how the food is going to affect our health and well being in this country.

Fruits and vegetables which are imported needs to be inspected by our inspector's to be certified as organic once it is established what is truly organic, by not lowering the standard, Or follows the laws of countries which have greatest number of healthy people like Switzerland for agricultures.

*At the least,* GMO food must be labeled so that people can have choices.

I believe it is idiotic to feed something (GMO foods, foods with insecticides and pesticides) to the population, our people, our brothers and sisters, our relatives and families, that is causing diseases that are hard to control and cure. We then have to spend a lot of money, our taxpayer money, pretending to fix them, when the problems are not fixable.

I would like to emphasize that in some foreign countries, GMO foods are not allowed to be sold in their markets or if allowed (all nations within European Unions= England, Scotland, Ireland, France, Italy, Germany, and Japan) in some, they are labeled GMO before they can be sold. As a result, the rate of health problems in England and Europe is much less. For instance, the rate of diabetes is around or less than 15 percent. In countries like Turkey and Switzerland, the rate is very low, less than 5 percent, for diabetes.

GMO food is affecting our workforce and the lives of our loved ones as well as our young men and women in the military, because at a very young age they are developing these conditions. This also means an increase in workers' compensation claims across the board, because with very trivial trauma our workers are going to have pain and suffer for a long time because they have lost the capacity to recover and heal. This will cause longer disabilities. Even when they stop working, they are not going to get better; their conditions will worsen with time.

The solution is *not* to treat them with pain medicine, called *pain management.*

When I look at the people in our Congress and Senators on television, from their faces it seems about 50 percent of them are already affected by these foods. They are getting symptomatic treatment. For the rest of them, it is only a matter of time until they are affected. At the same time, when I watch television and I see Queen Elizabeth being in her mid-eighties, with no health problems, but our last few presidents have had serious health problems, I wonder what is going on.

If you acquire any of the diseases mentioned above, how do you think it is going to affect your life?

If you are in pain, are you going to love your life or others?

If you cannot sleep, are in pain, and develop erectile dysfunction (ED), are you going to be in the mood for sex? If you develop blood pressure problems, most blood pressure medicines affect your sex drive, even if you do not have ED. Who is going to be happy? You, your husband, or your wife?

If you develop diabetes, a lot of problems come with it.

If you develop cancer or Alzheimer's, who is going to be happy?

If you have a child with Autism, mental retardation or any other problem who will be happy?

*So you see how our well being, happiness, love, enjoyment, and longevity are all related to the food we consume.*

*If we do not pay attention to this very important subject, do you know where we are heading?*

*We are on a self-destructive course. Money, gold, fame, and present medical science are not, and will not be, able to control or reverse the damages that already exist.*

*Let's hope the people in control and in decision-making roles come to their senses and see the bigger picture that is the future for our country.*

*Good luck to all of us.*

# About The Author

I am a student of science, dedicated to try and solve medical problems.

After six years of medical school and two years as a general medical officer, I continued my residency in medicine in Canada. To further my education, I continued in general surgery, and subsequently in orthopedic surgery. I have continued in medicine in the fields of orthopedic surgery, rheumatology, and endocrinology.

I am the fifth generation in my family to be a physician, and the last in my immediate family.

I grew up always knowing that I would be a doctor. My father used to say that the more you learn, the more you realize (the knowledge and science of the human body are very complicated), and that you never know enough. I realized during high school science classes that the human body works like a very complicated chemical machine.

Therefore, my understanding was that if I wanted to help my patients in the future, I needed to understand this complicated chemical factory, the human body. After high school, I started my undergraduate studies at the University of Rhode Island as a pre medicine and chemistry major. I had a great time at the University of Rhode Island and was very lucky to have dedicated professors.

At the time, my uncles Dr. John Yashar and Dr. James Yashar, both cardiovascular surgeons, were very persuasive to continue in Medicine. After a year, I realized through research that the University of Wisconsin in Madison had an excellent chemistry department. Therefore, after a year and a half at the University of Rhode Island, I transferred to the University of Wisconsin in Madison, to enroll in their chemistry department. I had the pleasure of knowing quite a few of the top people at the University of Wisconsin. I attended that university for a year and a half. At the time, I had the pleasure of learning about cloning, which was in progress and happening.

While I was at the University of Wisconsin in Madison, I was doing research for medical school. I had a meeting with the dean of the medical school and realized my dream was about to end. Since it was the height of the Vietnam era and there was a shortage of physicians, foreign students had no chance of getting into medical school, due to demands for American doctors was on the rise.

Therefore, with persuasion from my mother, I transferred to Pahlavi Medical School in Shiraz, Iran, which was affiliated with the University of Pennsylvania at the time. After six years of medical school and two years of military service as a general medical officer, I learned that a lot of people were in need of decent health care in the world. As a general medical officer, I served in remote areas to help people in villages. During my service to these people, I recognized that there are many people on the planet who are deprived of real medicine and hospitals.

Now I realize that people in remote villages were probably the healthiest on the planet, because the only problem they were facing was infectious diseases, which all responded to simple antibiotic treatments. There was an absence of any antibiotic resistance and MRSA among them. There was also an absence of cancer.

After finishing my military service, I arrived in the United States in April 1977 to start residency in general surgery. Unfortunately, I found out the hospital had lost what was called a j-1 slot, so I could not continue my education in medicine in the United States.

I took a trip to Canada, and with the help of Dr. Broomand and Kohanim, I started a year of residency in medicine at Kingston General Hospital in Kingston, Ontario, Canada. While I was in Kingston General Hospital in training, I learned that there was a prevalence of different problems in different geographic areas of the world. In Iran, there was mostly infectious diseases; and in Canada, there was autoimmune disorders, cardiovascular disease, and cancer.

After a year of medical residency, I arrived at the Jewish Hospital of Cincinnati in June 1978 for a year of general surgery. The next year, I was at the Bronx Lebanon Medical Center for another year of residency. Finally, in 1980, I started my lifelong wish of doing an orthopedic residency. I am grateful to Dr. Andrew Scheildhause; and to Dr. Andrew B. Weise, my chief of services at Bronx Lebanon Medical Center and University of Medicine and Dentistry of New Jersey.

# References

For more information, and references please refer to the following sites, magazines, and books:

Campbell's Operative Orthopedics

Civileats.com - March 28, 2011

Dangers of genetically engineered food

*Food, Inc.* by Peter Range

Google "GMO problems"

Life extension magazine

Kelley's Textbook of internal medicine

Organic Consumers Association

Orthopedic Knowledge Updates

responsibletechnology.org/healthcare-providers

Reuters.com - March 30, 2011

*Scientific American*, November 2011How food is absorbed

Scientific American: July2012, page 22, Bad for Bugs and Brains? (A common pesticide may interfere with a child's brain development)

Textbook of Harrisons

Textbook of Guyton physiology

The Journal of Musculoskeletal Medicine

*The Perricone Promise* by Dr. Nicholas Perricone

Washington manual for rheumatology

www.gmwatch.org - April 14, 2011

www.gmwatch.org-april 14/2012 BT TOXIN found in blood of- pregnant women

www.grist.org - April 12, 2011; March 29, 2011.

www.independent.co.uk-april 12,2012 GM maisze has polluted- rivers across the United States

www.latimes.com-April 12, 2011

www.latimes.com - April 04, 2011

www.responsibletechnology.org/blog/1340a - April 12, 2011

www.prnnewawire.com - April 07, 2011; March 30, 2011

www.psrast.org

www.prnnewawire.com - April 07, 2011; March 30, 2011

www.psrast.org

https://mail.google.com/mail/u/0/?shva=1#inbox/139543617f

http://naturalsociety.com/poland-ban-monsantos-genetically-modified-maize/

http://www.twnside.org.sg/title/furore-cn.htm

//www.google.com/#hl=en&sugexp=les%3B&gs_nf=1&gs_mss=letter%20of%20Japan%20to%20US%20on%20GM%20Soy&tok=QBJL UnlNpp0wPgyaQb5TFg&pq=lette

//www.google.com/#hl=en&sugexp=les%3B&gs_nf=1&gs_mss=gmo%20cant&to